Intermittent Fasting For Women

Intermittent Fasting For Women To Accelerate Fat Loss And Improve Health

Marie Richardson

Disclaimer

This Book has been written for information purposes only. Every effort has been made to make this Book as complete and accurate as possible. However, there may be mistakes in typography or content. Also, this Book provides information only up to the publishing date. Therefore, this Book should be used as a guide and not as the ultimate source.

Nothing in this Book should be considered, or used as a substitute for medical diagnosis, treatment, or advice. This Book do not constitute the practice of any medical professional advice, diagnosis or treatment. It is always best to talk to medical professionals for any questions regarding personal health or medical conditions. If there is a medical problem or condition, please contact a qualified medical professional immediately.

The purpose of this Book is to educate. The author and the publisher do not warrant that the information contained in this Book is fully complete and shall not be responsible for any errors or omissions. The author and publisher shall have neither liability nor responsibility to any person or entity with respect to any loss or damage caused or alleged to be caused directly or indirectly by this Book.

Table of Contents

Introduction

I want to thank you and congratulate you for buying the book, *"Intermittent Fasting For Women: An Easy To Follow Guide To Intermittent Fasting For Women To Accelerate Fat Loss And Improve Health"*.

This book contains proven steps and strategies on how to choose the right Intermittent Fasting Diet for you and apply it to your daily life.

Thanks again for buying this book, I hope you enjoy it!

Chapter 1: What is Intermittent Fasting?

Fasting has been part of human life throughout history. Our ancestors, who were hunter-gatherers, didn't have the luxury of markets, or the convenience of food storage facilities, or even have all-year-round food available. In our day-to-day lives, there are times when we couldn't find anything, or even find the time, to eat. Despite those moments, our bodies were able to function well. It seemed that our bodies have adapted well to extended periods of time without food, even though we're not consistently practicing fasting.

On the other hand, fasting is occasionally done due to people's religious beliefs. Major religions including Christianity, Buddhism, and Islam practice fasting on certain occasions. The truth is, occasional fasting is beneficial to our bodies and health. Because of this, fasting has been developed into a more "friendly" manner, so that it can be applied as a diet for weight loss – it's called the Intermittent Fasting Diet. Its revival and increasing popularity makes many wondering, what really is intermittent fasting? Is it safe for women? What are its benefits?

A Closer Look

Intermittent fasting, better known as IF, is a term used to describe a type of diet where individuals develop a pattern of food intake that cycle between periods of eating and not eating. Unlike many diets incessantly promoted today, an intermittent fasting diet does not focus on which foods that should be eaten while on a diet. Instead, it teaches us when to eat and when not to eat. It also teaches us that involving ourselves in this kind of diet is not a one-shot take. For it to be effective, it should be done constantly, and for life. In this respect, if applied properly, it can be more accurately described as a lifestyle.

What Does It Do To Your Body?

It's common knowledge that the human body cannot burn fat on its own unless we workout or do rigorous physical activities. This may come as a surprise. Fasting puts our bodies in a fat burning mode. Its main objective is weight loss. The question is how? To understand what intermittent fasting can do to our bodies, we must understand what happens to it first when we eat.

Food intake leads to digestion and absorption in our bodies. Typically, the food we eat lasts for 3 to 5 hours in our bodies – including digestion and absorption. During these hours, our bodies have high amounts of insulin which is a hormone released by our bodies to process glucose, or what we know as sugar. Majority of the food we eat today consists of carbohydrates which are converted to sugar in our bodies, thus the high insulin levels.

As soon as all food are digested and absorbed by the body, insulin levels start to go down because there's no more sugar to process. When there's little insulin in our bodies, it enters a fat-burning state. It's like a switch has been turned on to enable the body to burn fat on its own. There is a clearer explanation to how the body burns fat easily this way.

When there's food in our bodies and insulin levels are high, the body resorts to using the sugar and carbohydrates as its energy fuel. When insulin levels are low meanwhile, the body resorts to using fats as its source of energy. However, this only happens 8 to 12 hours after we eat and that's why in an intermittent fasting diet, not eating again within this time span is crucial. The most common duration for fasting is 16 hours, but there are many other variations. In Chapter 2, we'll discuss the most popular IF diets used today.

Why is Intermittent Fasting Popular Nowadays?

In 2012, a documentary by Dr. Michael Mosley on BBC Horizon introduced to the world a research by Dr. Krista Varady about Alternate Day Fasting (ADF). Since then, fasting took different forms from a wide range of sources. Two years later in 2014, Dr. Varady published her own book about her research where many has diverted from the real work she did. Today, because of the wide diversity of variations and IF's benefits, it has become a popular diet method for many. It especially catches the interest of people who are amazed at how our bodies can actually burn fat by itself.

Aside from burning fat easily, IF is popular because many find it convenient. During fasting days, you can just prepare black coffee and go to work. No need to prepare breakfast. No need to cleanup your mess in the kitchen. There's no delay for the day's activities ahead. As a result you become more productive. What's more, many IF practitioners find themselves energetic throughout the day, which increases productivity.

IF is also popular among people who eat snacks late in the evening because this diet allows it. It also allows you to eat whatever you want, as long as you are within your feeding period – more on that later. It literally offers us freedom to deal with our cravings during a limited period of time, rather than having to deal with them throughout the day and then give up and pig out.

In general, intermittent fasting is popular because it doesn't make people feel like they're on a diet because they're only setting a schedule for their feeding time.

This mindset makes IF more appealing and manageable. Let's look at more of its benefits to our health and body.

Chapter 2: Benefits of Intermittent Fasting

Weight loss is not the only reason why you should try intermittent fasting.

1. Intermittent fasting helps you look younger and live longer

Calorie restriction as a way to lengthen life is an accepted idea within the scientific community. It's because our bodies are wired for survival. When it is starving, it naturally finds ways to extend life and as a last resort, feeds itself. Yes, you read that right, but how?

Our liver feeds our body by producing glycogen, which is stored sugar or glucose. Glycogen helps nourish our bodies and keep them functioning until we eat again. In other words, intermittent fasting activates body mechanism for extending life. Various studies in the past have looked into this phenomenon.

In 1946, a study published in the Journal of Nutrition showed that IF prolonged life span of rats. To prove this even further, another study in 1983, this time published in the Journal of Gerontology (Gerontology is the study of the process of aging in humans), revealed that IF indeed does prolong life of lab rats. In a more recent study published in 2000, Japanese scientists from the Department of Psychosomatic Medicine in Kyushu University proved that repeated fasting influenced longevity of female mice.

Meanwhile, IF makes us look younger because it increases levels of growth hormone (HGH) in our blood. HGH is a protein-based hormone that stimulates cell regeneration and reproduction. A study in 1990 from the Medical College of Wisconsin, published in the New England Journal of Medicine, revealed that less GH levels is associated with rapid aging. This was also evident in another study done in 2002 by scientists from the John Hopkins University School of Medicine. Their research was published in the Journal of the American Medical Association.

2. Intermittent fasting helps you reduce stress

There are two ways on how IF can reduces stress in our lives. One is that it makes our lives simpler. As mentioned in Chapter 1, one of the reasons why IF is popular is because it makes mornings hassle-free. Without the need to eat breakfast on most days (this will depend on the variation of IF you'll use), you don't have to cook and prepare meals. You either drink water or black coffee, and then off you go to work.

Other meal times are also simpler because of IF. During fast days, most variations only require you to eat one major meal for a day. That means there's no need to worry or stress out on planning your next meals.

Second, IF reduces oxidative stress. We all know the harmful effects of free radicals in our bodies. It advances the aging process and makes our bodies highly prone to diseases and even cancer. We fight free radicals by eating foods rich in antioxidants. But did you know that there are certain antioxidants that can be found within our bodies? Yes, you got that right. Our bodies can naturally counteract harmful effects of free radicals.

However, due to limited production of natural antioxidants in our bodies, we experience oxidative stress. This is when our bodies cannot fight free radicals on its own. IF helps by enhancing our body's resistance to oxidative stress. A study from the National Institute on Aging's Intramural Research Program in 2005 revealed that IF reduces damages caused by oxidative and cellular stress. A more recent study in 2012, from the University of Hail in Saudi Arabia, backed up this claim by saying that intermittent fasting done during the season of Ramadan significantly reduced oxidative stress in their study subjects.

3. Intermittent fasting positively affects your hormones in a life-changing way

When the body receives no food for long periods of time, several things happen to it. Most significantly, hormone levels change that greatly affects the entire mechanism of our body. Hormonal changes happen because the body needs to make fat accessible when there are no other sources of energy to burn. Here are some of the major hormones that IF changes as it is applied to the body.

a. Insulin

According to Dr. Varady's research (mentioned in Chapter 1), IF significantly reduces insulin levels by 20-30%. We also discussed earlier that elevated levels of insulin makes it harder for our bodies to burn fat. Intermittent fasting also lowers blood sugar levels by 3-6%, reducing insulin resistance. It is that sad condition where the body produces insulin, but cannot use it effectively.

b. Human growth hormone (HGH)

HGH, a protein-based hormone, increases with IF. Aside from cell regeneration, high levels of this hormone further stimulate fat burning and promote muscle gain. In fact, when paired with exercise, IF can increase HGH by 2000% in men and 1300% in women.

c. Leptin and Ghrelin

Also known as the satiety hormone, Leptin regulates the body's feelings of hunger. Ghrelin, also known as the hunger hormone, signals the body when it is already hungry. These two play a major role in weight and appetite control. That is what a study from the VU University Medical Center in the Netherlands said in 2007. With intermittent fasting, both leptin and ghrelin are normalized.

4. Intermittent fasting protects the body against certain diseases and cancer

A study in 2010 from the Scripps Research Institute in California suggests that fasting induces autophagy. It is a normal bodily process where dysfunctional cells are destroyed to make way for new cell formation. In other words, IF helps the body to remove cellular waste, paving way for healthy cells to form. This in turn, protects the body against diseases and cancer. Prior to the Scripps research, a 2009 study from the University of Medicine and Dentistry of New Jersey stated that autophagy suppresses formation of tumors in the body.

In another scenario, cancer patients who undergo IF have shown less adverse effects of chemotherapy. Even better, patients who fasted before their treatment showed better chances of getting cured.

5. Intermittent fasting allows you to eat your favorite foods

This is a bonus. We can all enjoy intermittent fasting because it allows us to still eat the foods we love. With this in mind, it makes it easier to adapt to the diet. Many other diets fail because it's hard for practitioners to totally eliminate certain foods in their diet. What's more helpful is that when the body has fully adapted to IF, it doesn't become just another diet. It becomes part of your life. It becomes a lifestyle.

Ready to try it now? Let's take a look at some of the diet's popular variations.

Chapter 3: Different IF Methods

There are different methods of applying intermittent fasting to your diet. Here are the most popular methods available today.

The Leangains (16/8) Method: developed by Martin Berkhan

The Leangains method consists of 16 hours fasting and 8 hours feeding periods. It is named as it is because it is focused on gaining lean muscle. In other words, it involves serious fitness and strength training. Its rules on feeding put emphasis on the right nutrition for before and after workouts. It also involves strict macrocomposition and calorie cycling. However, Berkhan emphasized that meal timing is of utmost importance. Not maintaining a consistent feeding window throws our hormones abnormally.

A 2-day sample is shown below:

Day	AM					PM													AM					
Fast	7	8	9	10	11	12	1	2	3	4	5	6	7	8	9	10	11	12	1	2	3	4	5	6
Rest	7	8	9	10	11	12	1	2	3	4	5	6	7	8	9	10	11	12	1	2	3	4	5	6

*Red = fasting hours, Green = feeding hours

You'll see that in a typical fasting day, a person has an 8-hour feeding window from 12 noon until 7PM. During this time, a person can only eat the recommended daily calorie intake, where the last meal of the day consists of the largest percentage. For example:

12PM – lunch time 20-25% of daily calorie intake
2PM – snack 20-25% of daily calorie intake
6PM – dinner 50-60% of daily calorie intake

By 10PM, a person should already be sleeping because majority of the fasting period is spent this way. When a person wakes up at 7AM, workout should automatically follow after morning coffee (black only). Rest days are no different. However, no training or workout is involved during these days.

The Eat-Stop-Eat Method: developed by Brad Pilon

The Eat-Stop-Eat IF diet involves 24 hours of fasting for twice a week, at most. During fasting days, a person can drink water and other calorie-free drinks. During rest days, regular workouts must be implemented, especially resistance training. However, Pilon has not included meal and training recommendations (or specific workout routines) in his diet guidelines. Also, since there are no meal plans included, calorie counting and guidelines on macronutrients were not mentioned. Here is a 1-week sample:

D a y	AM			PM													AM					
F a s t		1	1	1									1	1	1							
	7 8 9 0 1	2	1 2 3 4 5 6 7 8 9 0	1	2	1 2 3 4 5 6																

R e s t				1	1	1										1	1	1							
	7	8	9	0	1	2	1	2	3	4	5	6	7	8	9	0	1	2	1	2	3	4	5	6
R e s t				1	1	1										1	1	1							
	7	8	9	0	1	2	1	2	3	4	5	6	7	8	9	0	1	2	1	2	3	4	5	6
R e s t				1	1	1										1	1	1							
	7	8	9	0	1	2	1	2	3	4	5	6	7	8	9	0	1	2	1	2	3	4	5	6
F a s t				1	1	1										1	1	1							
	7	8	9	0	1	2	1	2	3	4	5	6	7	8	9	0	1	2	1	2	3	4	5	6
R e s t				1	1	1										1	1	1							
	7	8	9	0	1	2	1	2	3	4	5	6	7	8	9	0	1	2	1	2	3	4	5	6
R e s t				1	1	1										1	1	1							
	7	8	9	0	1	2	1	2	3	4	5	6	7	8	9	0	1	2	1	2	3	4	5	6

In the Eat-Stop-Eat diet, you can eat regular meals 5 days a week, while fasting for 2 non-consecutive days.

The Warrior Diet (20/4): developed by Ori Hofmckler

The Warrior Diet involves 20 hours fasting and 4 hours feeding periods. For 20 hours, which is the "undereating" phase, a person can only drink water and calorie-free drinks. For the next 4 hours, which is the "overeating" phase, one large meal is allowed. This scheduling is based on Hofmekler's belief that our bodies can achieve and maintain ideal fitness levels if only we listen to its own biological, or circadian, clock. He believes that like our ancestors, we are naturally nocturnal eaters who eat one large meal at night before bed time.

During the undereating phase, a person is allowed to eat small meals. This is one of the reasons why many don't consider the Warrior Diet as an IF method. Small meals should only be composed of fresh juice, fruits, and raw vegetables. Small portions of protein are also allowed. During the overeating phase, a person can eat large servings of protein, vegetables, and fat. If a person is still hungry after eating, only then can carbohydrates be included in the meal.

Here is a 2-day sample:

Day	AM						PM												AM						
Fast	7	8	9	10	11	12	1	2	3	4	5	6	7	8	9	10	11	12	1	2	3	4	5	6
Fast	7	8	9	10	11	12	1	2	3	4	5	6	7	8	9	10	11	12	1	2	3	4	5	6

The Fat Loss Forever Method: developed by John Romaniello and Dan Go

The Fat Loss Forever method is a combination of guidelines based from the last three methods we discussed above. It consists of 1 day of fasting a week, which involves 36 hours of fasting followed by a cheat day. For the rest of the week, regular eating schedule is applied. Take a look at the 1-week sample below:

Day	AM						PM												AM					
Fast	7	8	9	10	11	12	1	2	3	4	5	6	7	8	9	10	11	12	1	2	3	4	5	6
Eat	7	8	9	10	11	12	1	2	3	4	5	6	7	8	9	10	11	12	1	2	3	4	5	6
Cheat	7	8	9	10	11	12	1	2	3	4	5	6	7	8	9	10	11	12	1	2	3	4	5	6
Reg lr	7	8	9	10	11	12	1	2	3	4	5	6	7	8	9	10	11	12	1	2	3	4	5	6
Reg lr	7	8	9	10	11	12	1	2	3	4	5	6	7	8	9	10	11	12	1	2	3	4	5	6
Reg lr	7	8	9	10	11	12	1	2	3	4	5	6	7	8	9	10	11	12	1	2	3	4	5	6
Reg lr	7	8	9	10	11	12	1	2	3	4	5	6	7	8	9	10	11	12	1	2	3	4	5	6

For regular days, different eating guidelines are provided. It also includes a weight training program for its practitioners.

The Fast Diet (5/2): developed by Michael Mosley

We discussed Dr. Michael Mosley in Chapter 1. After his interview with Dr. Krista Varady, he started his own method of intermittent fasting, the Fast Diet. It involves regular feeding for 5 days and fasting for 2 non-consecutive days. Compared to all the other diets we discussed, many find this method IF easier to adhere to. Here is a 1-week sample:

Day	AM						PM											AM						
Fast	7	8	9	10	11	12	1	2	3	4	5	6	7	8	9	10	11	12	1	2	3	4	5	6
Reglr	7	8	9	10	11	12	1	2	3	4	5	6	7	8	9	10	11	12	1	2	3	4	5	6
Reglr	7	8	9	10	11	12	1	2	3	4	5	6	7	8	9	10	11	12	1	2	3	4	5	6
Reglr	7	8	9	10	11	12	1	2	3	4	5	6	7	8	9	10	11	12	1	2	3	4	5	6
Fast	7	8	9	10	11	12	1	2	3	4	5	6	7	8	9	10	11	12	1	2	3	4	5	6
Reglr	7	8	9	10	11	12	1	2	3	4	5	6	7	8	9	10	11	12	1	2	3	4	5	6
Reglr	7	8	9	10	11	12	1	2	3	4	5	6	7	8	9	10	11	12	1	2	3	4	5	6

For fasting days, practitioners can eat 2-3 small meals throughout the day. Meals for these days should only have a total of 500 calories for men and 600 calories for women. For regular days, practitioners can eat normally again.

The UpDayDownDay Diet: developed James Johnson

The UpDayDownDay diet, also known as the Alternate-Day Diet, is similar to the Fast Diet. During "up" days, a person can eat a meal with a total of calories that are recommended for daily intake. During "down days," a person can only get to eat meals with a total of 400-500 calories. Here is a 1-week sample:

Day	AM					PM												AM						
Fast	7	8	9	10	11	12	1	2	3	4	5	6	7	8	9	10	11	12	1	2	3	4	5	6
Reglr	7	8	9	10	11	12	1	2	3	4	5	6	7	8	9	10	11	12	1	2	3	4	5	6
Fast	7	8	9	10	11	12	1	2	3	4	5	6	7	8	9	10	11	12	1	2	3	4	5	6
Reglr	7	8	9	10	11	12	1	2	3	4	5	6	7	8	9	10	11	12	1	2	3	4	5	6
Fast	7	8	9	10	11	12	1	2	3	4	5	6	7	8	9	10	11	12	1	2	3	4	5	6
Reglr	7	8	9	10	11	12	1	2	3	4	5	6	7	8	9	10	11	12	1	2	3	4	5	6
Fast	7	8	9	10	11	12	1	2	3	4	5	6	7	8	9	10	11	12	1	2	3	4	5	6

The Fast 5 Diet (19/5): developed by Bert Herring

The Fast Diet includes 19 hours of fasting and 5 hours of feeding periods. During fasting hours, dieters are only allowed water and calorie-free drinks. During feeding hours, dieters can eat any food as long as they are healthy to the body. Keep away from highly-processed foods. Here is a 2-day sample of a Fast 5 schedule:

Day	AM					PM												AM						
Fast	7	8	9	10	11	12	1	2	3	4	5	6	7	8	9	10	11	12	1	2	3	4	5	6
Fast	7	8	9	10	11	12	1	2	3	4	5	6	7	8	9	10	11	12	1	2	3	4	5	6

It's not hard to see that these methods should be regularly practiced once applied. They become part of life, not just a passing fancy. Doctors and fitness experts who developed these methods are serious about their goals which is weight loss. However, in order for these diets to become more effective and enable us to maintain a healthy weight, these diets must become part of our lifestyles.

What IF Method to Choose?

Knowing these methods, one question remain: what IF method should you choose? Here's a tip: listen to your body. All our bodies are different from one another. Consider the guidelines for each method as a deciding factor. Will it create conflict with your schedule? What is most convenient for you? Are you comfortable counting your calorie intake with each meal? What is your fitness goal? Use these questions when choosing the right IF method.

When IF is not Allowed

Please be guided that any form of intermittent fasting is not allowed when a woman is

Pregnant

Many changes occur in a woman's body when she's pregnant. Along with these changes, certain nutritional needs are needed more during this time. IF can disrupt these changes and needs thus, IF is not suitable for pregnant women.

Suffering from an eating disorder, or has a history of eating disorder

Intermittent fasting is not allowed for women with history of eating disorder, which means, it is also not allowed for women suffering from it. IF can create further health problems if applied.

Sleep-deprived or having trouble getting enough sleep, and chronically stressed

Without enough sleep and with too much stress, the body becomes weak and unable to function well. Before going through IF, the body must be ready and strong.

New to diet and exercise

It's better if women know the basics of nutrition and exercise before implementing an IF lifestyle. Better yet, consult a doctor first.

When intermittent fasting is not allowed, there's no reason to be sad. This is a perfect time to learn the fundamentals of good nutrition, which is the basic foundation of our health and fitness. Good nutrition involves eating healthy whole foods, exercising regularly, and staying consistent with fitness goals.

On the other hand, for women who have chosen the IF path, here are some reminders. Stop fasting if the following changes occur:

- Irregular menstrual cycle or the absence of it
- Difficulty sleeping
- Hair falling out in substantial amount
- Acne or dry skin starts to develop
- Irregular heartbeat or palpitations
- Painful sexual intercourse
- Intense mood swings
- High-sensitivity to stress and cold weather
- Noticeable slow digestion or bloating
- Always unusually tired, especially after workouts

IF may be popular and many people use it, especially men, but women's bodies are different from them. Women's bodies have different needs. Again, listen to it.

Chapter 4: Starting Your First Fast

Even just thinking about intermittent fasting is overwhelming enough. Applying it to our lifestyles and going through it is another thing. To help you get started, here are some important tips that can help you start your IF diet.

Take it Slow

Let's take the Leangains (16/8) method as an example. At first, many women find it hard to adhere to the 16 hours without food. Women are wired to be highly sensitive to signals of hunger. Our bodies respond to leptin and ghrelin differently than men. To make Leangains easier, and for the sake of our hunger, shorten the time of fasting at first. Take a look at the sample below:

Day	AM					PM												AM						
Fast	7	8	9	10	11	12	1	2	3	4	5	6	7	8	9	10	11	12	1	2	3	4	5	6
Rest	7	8	9	10	11	12	1	2	3	4	5	6	7	8	9	10	11	12	1	2	3	4	5	6
Fast	7	8	9	10	11	12	1	2	3	4	5	6	7	8	9	10	11	12	1	2	3	4	5	6
Rest	7	8	9	10	11	12	1	2	3	4	5	6	7	8	9	10	11	12	1	2	3	4	5	6
Fas	7	8	9	10	11	12	1	2	3	4	5	6	7	8	9	10	11	12	1	2	3	4	5	6

t R e s t	7	8	9	10	11	12	1	2	3	4	5	6	7	8	9	10	11	12	1	2	3	4	5	6
F a s t	7	8	9	10	11	12	1	2	3	4	5	6	7	8	9	10	11	12	1	2	3	4	5	6

In the span of 1 week, the feeding window is reduced every day until it reached the targeted 8 hours. This can be helpful for women who feel hungry all the time (don't worry, it's normal). This tip can be used to adjust gradually to the meal scheduling that IF requires.

Sleep it Off

The great thing about IF is that hunger pangs can be prevented by sleeping during the majority of the fasting period. It is crucial for IF dieters to sleep amply, that's why women with sleeping problems are not allowed to use IF dieting. By sleeping during fasting hours, there's less pressure to eat and more time for the body to rest and regain energy. Let's use the sample above again to demonstrate the sleeping pattern of a dieter under the Leangains diet.

D a y	AM					PM												AM					
F a s t	7	8	9	10	11	12	1	2	3	4	5	6	7	8	9	10	11	12	1	2	3	4	5	6
R e s t	7	8	9	10	11	12	1	2	3	4	5	6	7	8	9	10	11	12	1	2	3	4	5	6
F a s t	7	8	9	10	11	12	1	2	3	4	5	6	7	8	9	10	11	12	1	2	3	4	5	6
R e s	7	8	9	10	11	12	1	2	3	4	5	6	7	8	9	10	11	12	1	2	3	4	5	6

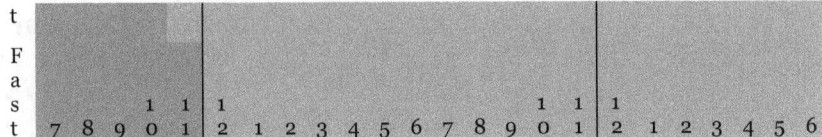

The red area signifies the fasting hours, while the gray area signifies sleeping hours. Notice how many number of hours sleeping takes compared to the fasting hours. If fasting is done during the day, when a person is wide awake, it might be harder to accomplish fasting hours because our body will automatically signal us to eat.

Never Do It at Two

Do not fast for two consecutive days or twice in a week. Remember, intermittent fasting involves calorie restriction. There are days when the recommended calorie intake is not reached. By adding one more day to that can further reduce calorie intake by an additional 30%. This leads to lack of energy and strength. It can also worsen hunger pangs, which causes over-eating.

Water is Your Friend

In an IF diet, water is your new best friend. An empty stomach can make us feel hungry easier and faster, so drink lots of water during fasting hours. Other beverages are also allowed, but avoid carbonated and sugary drinks. Plain tea and coffee are also recommended, but drink them only at daytime so as not to disrupt sleeping pattern.

More Tips

- Do not exercise on fasting days. Reserve energy. Otherwise, you'll feel hungry faster.

- Eat fresh, whole foods only. Processed foods only bring havoc to our hormones and affect our metabolism negatively.
- Make IF easier by changing your perspective about it. Pilon, author of Eat Stop Eat diet (mentioned in Chapter 3), says that it can help to think about IF as a break or rest from eating. This is especially true with today's overeating trend.
- Try intermittent fasting for two months before deciding whether it is truly suitable or not. It is during this time that the effects of IF can be seen and felt, though the first week of fasting is life-changing enough.

Lastly, do not be afraid to try IF out. Many stories about losing muscle and strength come out about IF. It's not true. Otherwise, why would IF methods such as Leangains and the Warrior Diet be successful? Workouts are major parts of these IF diets.

Conclusion

Thank you again for buying this book!

I hope this book was able to help you to understand intermittent fasting better and let you decide to try it out.

The next step is to choose one method of IF and use it. Follow the tips mentioned for an easier IF dieting.

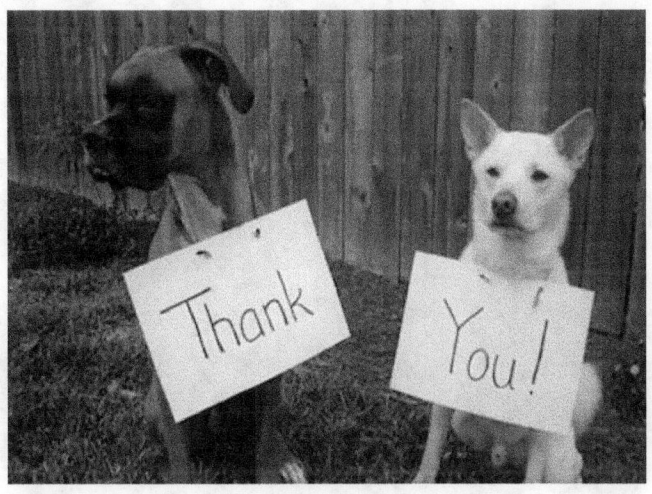

Finally, if you enjoyed this book, then I'd like to ask you for a favor, would you be kind enough to leave a review for this book on Amazon? It'd be greatly appreciated!

Thank you and good luck!

www.ingramcontent.com/pod-product-compliance
Lightning Source LLC
Chambersburg PA
CBHW061944280526
45787CB00004B/1714